Heart Healthy Home Cooking
African American Style

With Every Heartbeat Is Life

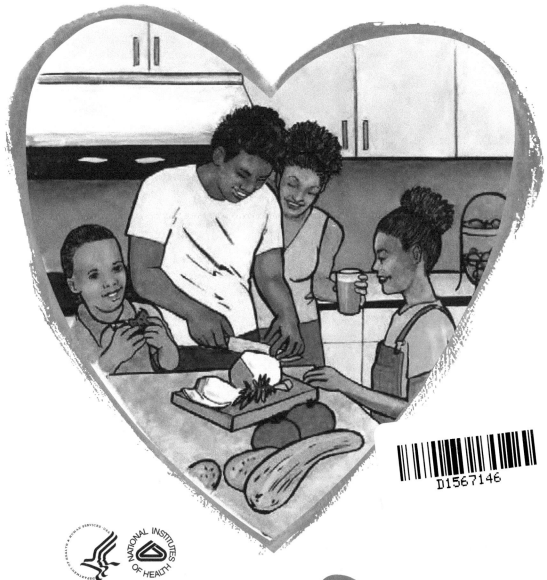

U.S. Department of Health and Human Services
National Institutes of Health

National **Heart**
Lung and Blood Institute

NIH Publication No. 08-3792
Revised May 2008

Published by Books Express Publishing
Copyright © Books Express, 2012
ISBN 978-1-78266-073-6

Books Express publications are available from all good retail and online booksellers. For
publishing proposals and direct ordering please contact us at: info@books-express.com

Special thanks to Wahida Karmally, Dr.P.H., R.D., CDE, CLS, and her colleagues at the Irving Center for Research at Columbia University for testing the recipes with the African American community.

Recipes were analyzed using the Nutrition Data System for Research, 2005.

Table of Contents

Introduction

Salads, Vegetables, and Side Dishes

Good-for-You Cornbread 4

Homestyle Biscuits 5

Savory Potato Salad 6

Candied Yams 7

Smothered Greens 8

Limas and Spinach 9

Vegetable Stew 10

Classic Macaroni and Cheese 11

Autumn Salad 12

Flavorful Green Beans 13

Caribbean Casserole 14

Spicy Okra 15

Main Dishes

Crispy Oven-Fried Chicken 18

Mouth-Watering Oven-Fried Fish 19

Finger-Licking Curried Chicken 20

Poached Salmon 21

Jamaican Jerk Chicken... 22

Baked Pork Chops 23

Jumpin' Jambalaya.. 24

Scrumptious Meat Loaf 25

Spicy Southern Barbecued Chicken.. 26

Desserts

1-2-3 Peach Cobbler 28

Mock-Southern Sweet Potato Pie 29

Southern Banana Pudding 30

Summer Breeze Smoothie 31

Tangy Fruit Salad 32

Recipe Substitutions for Heart Healthy Cooking

.... 34

Is It Done Yet? Temperature Rules for Safe Cooking

.... 36

Introduction

Good food is one of life's great joys. And good meals are a shared pleasure at the heart of African American family life and special celebrations. This recipe book brings together many African American favorite recipes, prepared in a heart healthy way, lower in saturated fat, cholesterol, and sodium! It shows how to prepare dishes in ways that help protect you and your family from heart disease and stroke. This is important because heart disease and stroke are the first and the third leading cause of death for African Americans. By making small changes in the way you and your family eat, you can help reduce your risk for heart disease and stroke.

This updated recipe book includes new recipes, along with some of your old favorites. New information on heart healthy food substitutions and food safety is also included.

So, make a start today. Give those old favorites a new, tasty, heart healthy makeover. And help keep the heart of your family strong!

Salads, Vegetables, and Side Dishes

Good-for-You Cornbread

Homestyle Biscuits

Savory Potato Salad

Candied Yams

Smothered Greens

Limas and Spinach

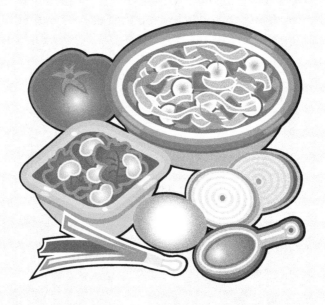

Vegetable Stew

Classic Macaroni and Cheese

Autumn Salad

Flavorful Green Beans

Caribbean Casserole

Spicy Okra

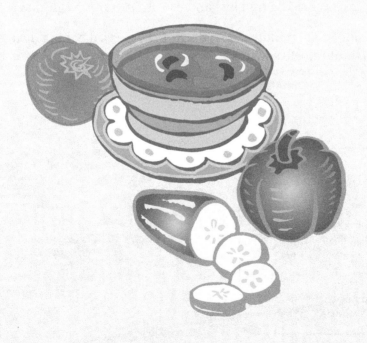

Good-for-You Cornbread

This is not only good *for* you, but good *in* you—making it a healthy comfort food.

- 1 cup cornmeal
- 1 cup flour
- ¼ cup sugar
- 1 teaspoon baking powder
- 1 cup low-fat (1%) buttermilk
- 1 egg, whole
- ¼ cup margarine, regular, tub
- 1 teaspoon vegetable oil (to grease baking pan)

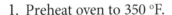

1. Preheat oven to 350 °F.

2. Mix together cornmeal, flour, sugar, and baking powder.

3. In another bowl, combine buttermilk and egg. Beat lightly.

4. Slowly add buttermilk and egg mixture to dry ingredients.

5. Add margarine and mix by hand or with mixer for 1 minute.

6. Bake for 20–25 minutes in an 8 x 8-inch, greased baking dish. Cool. Cut into 10 squares.

Yield:	**10 servings**
Serving size:	**1 square**
Calories	178
Total Fat	6 g
Saturated Fat	1 g
Cholesterol	22 mg
Sodium	94 mg
Total Fiber	1 g
Protein	4 g
Carbohydrates	27 g
Potassium	132 mg

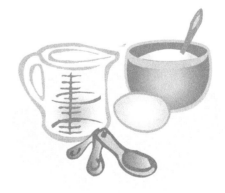

Homestyle Biscuits

Update your homestyle biscuits with this easy, low-fat recipe.

- **2 cups all purpose flour**
- **2 teaspoons baking powder**
- **¼ teaspoon baking soda**
- **¼ teaspoon salt**
- **2 tablespoons sugar**
- **⅔ cup low-fat (1%) buttermilk**
- **3 tablespoons + 1 teaspoon vegetable oil**

1. Preheat oven to 450 °F.

2. In medium bowl, combine flour, baking powder, baking soda, salt, and sugar.

3. In small bowl, stir together buttermilk and oil. Pour over flour mixture and stir until well mixed.

4. On lightly floured surface, knead dough gently for 10–12 strokes. Roll or pat dough to ¾-inch thickness. Cut with a 2-inch round biscuit or cookie cutter, dipping cookie cutter in flour between cuts. Transfer biscuits to an ungreased baking sheet.

5. Bake for 12 minutes or until golden brown. Serve warm.

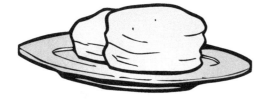

Yield:	**15 servings**
Serving size:	**1 biscuit**
Calories	99
Total Fat	3 g
Saturated Fat	0 g
Cholesterol	0 mg
Sodium	72 mg
Total Fiber	1 g
Protein	2 g
Carbohydrates	15 g
Potassium	102 mg

Savory Potato Salad

Here's a potato salad that's both traditional and new—with great taste and a low-fat twist.

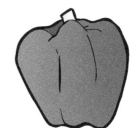

- 6 medium potatoes (about 2 pounds)
- 2 stalks celery, finely chopped
- 2 scallions, finely chopped
- ¼ cup red bell pepper, coarsely chopped
- ¼ cup green bell pepper, coarsely chopped
- 1 tablespoon onion, finely chopped
- 1 egg, hard boiled, chopped
- 6 tablespoons mayonnaise, light
- 1 teaspoon mustard
- ½ teaspoon salt
- ¼ teaspoon black pepper
- ¼ teaspoon dill weed, dried

1. Wash potatoes, cut in half, and place in saucepan of cold water.

2. Cook covered over medium heat for 25–30 minutes or until tender.

3. Drain and dice potatoes when cool.

4. Add vegetables and egg to potatoes and toss.

5. Blend together mayonnaise, mustard, salt, pepper, and dill weed.

6. Pour dressing over potato mixture and stir gently to coat evenly.

7. Chill for at least 1 hour before serving.

Yield:	**10 servings**
Serving size:	**½ cup**
Calories	98
Total Fat	2 g
Saturated Fat	0 g
Cholesterol	21 mg
Sodium	212 mg
Total Fiber	2 g
Protein	2 g
Carbohydrates	18 g
Potassium	291 mg

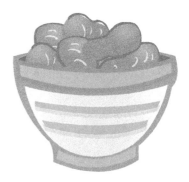

Candied Yams

A bit of margarine and some orange juice make this dish sweet.

- 3 medium yams (1½ cups)
- ¼ cup brown sugar, packed
- 1 teaspoon flour, sifted
- ¼ teaspoon salt
- ¼ teaspoon ground cinnamon
- ¼ teaspoon ground nutmeg
- ¼ teaspoon orange peel
- 1 teaspoon soft tub margarine
- ½ cup orange juice

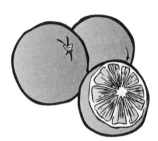

1. Preheat oven to 350 °F.

2. Cut yams in half and boil until tender, but firm (about 20 minutes). When cool enough to handle, peel and slice into ¼-inch thickness.

3. Combine sugar, flour, salt, cinnamon, nutmeg, and grated orange peel.

4. Place half of sliced yams in medium-sized casserole dish. Sprinkle with spiced sugar mixture.

5. Dot with half the amount of margarine.

6. Add second layer of yams, using the rest of the ingredients in the order above. Add orange juice.

7. Bake uncovered for 20 minutes.

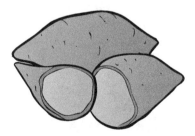

Yield:	6 servings
Serving size:	¼ cup
Calories	110
Total Fat	0 g
Saturated Fat	0 g
Cholesterol	0 mg
Sodium	115 mg
Total Fiber	2 g
Protein	1 g
Carbohydrates	25 g
Potassium	344 mg

Smothered Greens

These healthy greens get their rich flavor from smoked turkey, instead of fatback.

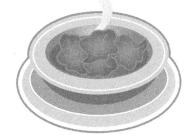

- 3 cups water
- ¼ pound smoked turkey breast, skinless
- 1 tablespoon fresh hot pepper, chopped
- ¼ teaspoon cayenne pepper
- ¼ teaspoon cloves, ground
- 2 cloves garlic, crushed
- ½ teaspoon thyme
- 1 scallion, chopped
- 1 teaspoon ginger, ground
- ¼ cup onion, chopped
- 2 pounds greens (mustard, turnip, collard, kale, or mixture)

1. Place all ingredients except greens into large saucepan and bring to boil.

2. Prepare greens by washing thoroughly and removing stems.

3. Tear or slice leaves into bite-size pieces.

4. Add greens to turkey stock. Cook for 20–30 minutes until tender.

Yield:	5 servings
Serving size:	1 cup
Calories	80
Total Fat	2 g
Saturated Fat	0 g
Cholesterol	16 mg
Sodium	378 mg
Total Fiber	4 g
Protein	9 g
Carbohydrates	9 g
Potassium	472 mg

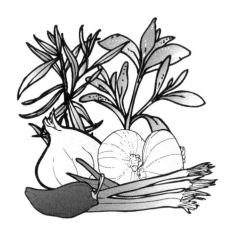

Limas and Spinach

Your family will love vegetables cooked this way.

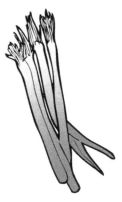

- 2 cups frozen lima beans
- 1 tablespoon vegetable oil
- 1 cup fennel, cut in 4-inch strips
- ½ cup onion, chopped
- ¼ cup low-sodium chicken broth
- 4 cups leaf spinach, washed thoroughly
- 1 tablespoon distilled vinegar
- ⅛ teaspoon black pepper
- 1 tablespoon raw chives

1. Steam or boil lima beans in unsalted water for about 10 minutes. Drain.

2. In skillet, saute onions and fennel in oil.

3. Add beans and broth to onions and cover. Cook for 2 minutes.

4. Stir in spinach. Cover and cook until spinach has wilted, about 2 minutes.

5. Stir in vinegar and pepper. Cover and let stand for 30 seconds.

6. Sprinkle with chives and serve.

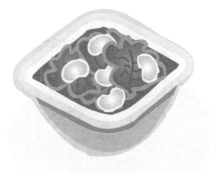

Yield:	7 servings
Serving size:	½ cup
Calories	93
Total Fat	2 g
Saturated Fat	0 g
Cholesterol	0 mg
Sodium	84 mg
Total Fiber	6 g
Protein	5 g
Carbohydrates	15 g
Potassium	452 mg

Vegetable Stew

Here's a great new way to use summer vegetables.

- 3 cups water
- 1 cube vegetable bouillon, low sodium
- 2 cups white potatoes, cut in 2-inch strips
- 2 cups carrots, sliced
- 4 cups summer squash, cut in 1-inch squares
- 1 cup summer squash, cut in 4 chunks
- 1 15-ounce can sweet corn, rinsed and drained (or 2 ears fresh corn, 1½ cups)
- 1 teaspoon thyme
- 2 cloves garlic, minced
- 1 stalk scallion, chopped
- ½ small hot pepper, chopped
- 1 cup onion, coarsely chopped
- 1 cup tomatoes, diced

Note: You can add other favorite vegetables, such as broccoli and cauliflower.

1. Put water and bouillon in large pot and bring to a boil.

2. Add potatoes and carrots and simmer for 5 minutes.

3. Add remaining ingredients, except for tomatoes, and continue cooking for 15 minutes over medium heat.

4. Remove 4 chunks of squash and puree in blender.

5. Return pureed mixture to pot and let cook for 10 minutes more.

6. Add tomatoes and cook for another 5 minutes.

7. Remove from heat and let sit for 10 minutes to allow stew to thicken.

Yield:	**8 servings**
Serving size:	**1¼ cup**
Calories	119
Total Fat	1 g
Saturated Fat	0 g
Cholesterol	0 mg
Sodium	196 mg
Total Fiber	4 g
Protein	4 g
Carbohydrates	27 g
Potassium	524 mg

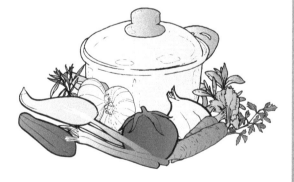

Classic Macaroni and Cheese

This recipe proves you don't have to give up your favorite dishes to eat heart healthy meals. Here's a lower-fat version of a true classic.

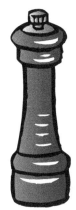

- 2 cups macaroni
- 2 cups onions, chopped
- 2 cups evaporated fat-free milk
- 1 medium egg, beaten
- ¼ teaspoon black pepper
- 1¼ cups low-fat cheddar cheese, finely shredded
- nonstick cooking spray, as needed

1. Cook macaroni according to directions—but do not add salt to the cooking water. Drain and set aside.

2. Spray casserole dish with nonstick cooking spray.

3. Preheat oven to 350 °F.

4. Lightly spray saucepan with nonstick cooking spray. Add onions to saucepan and saute for about 3 minutes.

5. In another bowl, combine macaroni, onions, and the rest of the ingredients and mix thoroughly.

6. Transfer mixture into casserole dish.

7. Bake for 25 minutes or until bubbly. Let stand for 10 minutes before serving.

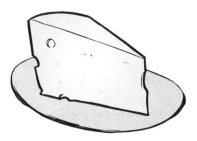

Yield:	8 servings
Serving size:	½ cup
Calories	200
Total Fat	4 g
Saturated Fat	2 g
Cholesterol	34 mg
Sodium	120 mg
Total Fiber	1 g
Protein	11 g
Carbohydrates	29 g
Potassium	119 mg

Autumn Salad

This fresh and tasty salad will delight all.

- 1 medium Granny Smith apple, sliced thinly (with skin)
- 2 tablespoons lemon juice
- 1 bag (about 5 cups) mixed lettuce greens (or your favorite lettuce)
- ½ cup dried cranberries
- ¼ cup walnuts, chopped
- ¼ cup unsalted sunflower seeds
- ⅓ cup low-fat raspberry vinaigrette dressing

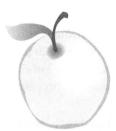

1. Sprinkle lemon juice on the apple slices.

2. Mix the lettuce, cranberries, apple, walnuts, and sunflower seeds in a bowl.

3. Toss with ⅓ cup of raspberry vinaigrette dressing, to lightly cover the salad.

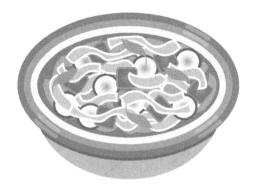

Yield:	**6 servings**
Serving size:	**1 cup**
Calories	138
Total Fat	7 g
Saturated Fat	1 g
Cholesterol	0 mg
Sodium	41 mg
Total Fiber	3 g
Protein	3 g
Carbohydrates	19 g
Potassium	230 mg

Flavorful Green Beans

The seasonings are perfect companions to the green beans.

- **2 pounds fresh green beans**
- **½ cup water**
- **⅓ cup onions, chopped**
- **4 cloves garlic, chopped**
- **nonstick cooking spray**
- **½ teaspoon black pepper**
- **½ teaspoon dried basil**
- **½ teaspoon oregano**

1. Rinse green beans and snap off tips.

2. Place green beans in a large pot and add ½ cup of cold water.

3. Cook green beans on stovetop over medium heat for 10 minutes.

4. In a separate pan, saute chopped onions and garlic, using the cooking spray, for 5 minutes or until they are tender and very lightly browned.

5. Add onions, garlic, and black pepper to green beans. Spray the cooking spray over mixture, and cook on medium heat for another 20 minutes or until green beans are tender, but not soft. Stir occasionally.

6. Sprinkle dried basil and oregano over green beans. Mix and serve.

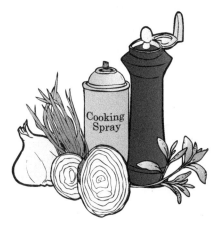

Yield:	7 servings
Serving size:	**1 cup**
Calories	40
Total Fat	0 g
Saturated Fat	0 g
Cholesterol	0 mg
Sodium	12 mg
Total Fiber	4 g
Protein	2 g
Carbohydrates	9 g
Potassium	179 mg

Caribbean Casserole

This tropical-inspired dish is gently spiced for a rich flavor.

- 1 medium onion, chopped
- ½ green pepper, diced
- 1 tablespoon canola oil
- 1 14½-ounce can stewed tomatoes
- 1 16-ounce can black beans (or beans of your choice)
- 1 teaspoon oregano leaves
- ½ teaspoon garlic powder
- 1½ cups instant brown rice, uncooked

1. Saute onion and green pepper in canola oil, in a large pan, until tender. Do not brown.

2. Add tomatoes, beans (include liquid from both), oregano, and garlic powder. Bring to a boil. Stir in rice and cover. Reduce heat to simmer for 5 minutes. Remove from heat and let stand for 5 minutes.

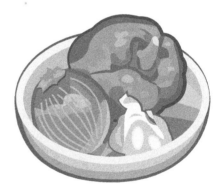

Yield:	**10 servings**
Serving size:	**1 cup**
Calories	185
Total Fat	1 g
Saturated Fat	0 g
Cholesterol	0 mg
Sodium	297 mg
Total Fiber	7 g
Protein	7 g
Carbohydrates	37 g
Potassium	292 mg

Spicy Okra

You will love this zesty okra dish.

- 2 10-ounce packages frozen, cut okra
- 1 tablespoon vegetable oil
- 1 medium onion, coarsely chopped
- 1 14½-ounce can of diced tomatoes
- 1 fresh jalapeño pepper (or habanero chile), pierced 3 times with a fork
- ½ teaspoon salt
- ¼ teaspoon black pepper

1. Rinse okra in a colander under hot water.

2. Heat oil in a 10-inch heavy skillet over moderately high heat. Saute onion for about 3 minutes. Add tomatoes (including juice) and chile, and boil. Stir the mixture for 8 minutes. Add okra and cook, gently stirring, until okra is tender, about 5 minutes.

3. Stir in salt and pepper and discard the chile.

Yield:	10 servings
Serving size:	½ cup
Calories	99
Total Fat	4 g
Saturated Fat	1 g
Cholesterol	0 mg
Sodium	133 mg
Total Fiber	5 g
Protein	4 g
Carbohydrates	15 g
Potassium	563 mg

Main Dishes

Crispy Oven-Fried Chicken

Mouth-Watering Oven-Fried Fish

Finger-Licking Curried Chicken

Poached Salmon

Jamaican Jerk Chicken

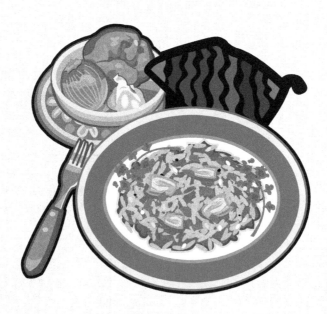

Baked Pork Chops

Jumpin' Jambalaya

Scrumptious Meat Loaf

Spicy Southern Barbecued Chicken

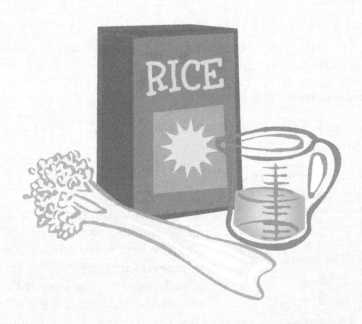

Crispy Oven-Fried Chicken

Kids will love this chicken—and it's good for the heart.

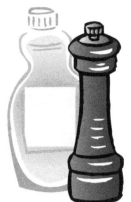

- ½ cup fat-free milk or buttermilk
- 1 teaspoon poultry seasoning
- 1 cup cornflakes, crumbled
- 1½ tablespoons onion powder
- 1½ tablespoons garlic powder
- 2 teaspoons black pepper
- 2 teaspoons dried hot pepper, crushed
- 1 teaspoon ginger, ground
- 8 pieces chicken, skinless (4 breasts, 4 drumsticks)
- a few shakes paprika
- 1 teaspoon vegetable oil

1. Preheat oven to 350 °F.

2. Add ½ teaspoon of poultry seasoning to milk.

3. Combine all other spices with cornflake crumbs, and place in plastic bag.

4. Wash chicken and pat dry. Dip chicken into milk and shake to remove excess. Quickly shake in bag with seasonings and crumbs, and remove the chicken from the bag.

5. Refrigerate chicken for 1 hour.

6. Remove chicken from refrigerator and sprinkle lightly with paprika for color.

7. Space chicken evenly on greased baking pan.

8. Cover with aluminum foil and bake for 40 minutes. Remove foil and continue baking for another 30–40 minutes or until meat can easily be pulled away from the bone with fork. Drumsticks may require less baking time than breasts. Crumbs will form crispy "skin."

Yield:	10 servings
Serving size:	½ breast or 2 small drumsticks
Calories	117
Total Fat	3 g
Saturated Fat	1 g
Cholesterol	49 mg
Sodium	67 mg
Total Fiber	1 g
Protein	17 g
Carbohydrates	6 g
Potassium	1 mg

Note: Do not turn chicken during baking.

Mouth-Watering Oven-Fried Fish

This heart healthy dish can be made with many kinds of fish—to be enjoyed over and over.

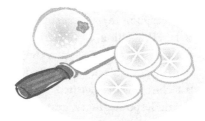

- 2 pounds fish fillets
- 1 tablespoon lemon juice, fresh
- ¼ cup fat-free or 1% buttermilk
- 2 drops hot sauce
- 1 teaspoon fresh garlic, minced
- ¼ teaspoon white pepper, ground
- ¼ teaspoon salt
- ¼ teaspoon onion powder
- ½ cup cornflakes, crumbled, or regular bread crumbs
- 1 tablespoon vegetable oil
- 1 fresh lemon, cut in wedges

1. Preheat oven to 475 °F.

2. Clean and rinse fish. Wipe fillets with lemon juice and pat dry.

3. Combine milk, hot sauce, and garlic.

4. Combine pepper, salt, and onion powder with crumbs and place on plate.

5. Let fillets sit briefly in milk. Remove and coat fillets on both sides with seasoned crumbs. Let stand briefly until coating sticks to each side of fish.

6. Arrange on lightly oiled shallow baking dish.

7. Bake for 20 minutes on middle rack without turning.

8. Cut into 6 pieces. Serve with fresh lemon.

Yield:	6 servings
Serving size:	1 cut piece
Calories	183
Total Fat	2 g
Saturated Fat	0 g
Cholesterol	80 mg
Sodium	325 mg
Total Fiber	1 g
Protein	30 g
Carbohydrates	10 g
Potassium	453 mg

Finger-Licking Curried Chicken

The name tells all—ginger and curry powder make it irresistible.

- 1½ teaspoons curry powder
- 1 teaspoon thyme, crushed
- 1 stalk scallion, chopped
- 1 tablespoon hot pepper, chopped
- 1 teaspoon black pepper, ground
- 8 cloves garlic, crushed
- 1 tablespoon ginger, grated
- ¾ teaspoon salt
- 8 pieces chicken, skinless (4 breasts, 4 drumsticks)
- 1 tablespoon olive oil
- 1 cup water
- 1 medium white potato, diced
- 1 large onion, chopped

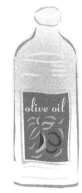

1. Wash chicken and pat dry.

2. Mix together curry powder, thyme, scallion, hot pepper, cayenne pepper, black pepper, garlic, ginger, and salt.

3. Sprinkle seasoning mixture on chicken.

4. Marinate for at least 2 hours in refrigerator.

5. Heat oil in skillet over medium heat. Add chicken and saute.

6. Add water and allow chicken to cook over medium heat for 30 minutes.

7. Add diced potatoes and cook for an additional 30 minutes.

8. Add onions and cook for 15 minutes more or until meat is tender.

Yield:	10 servings
Serving size:	½ breast or 2 small drumsticks
Calories	134
Total Fat	4 g
Saturated Fat	1 g
Cholesterol	49 mg
Sodium	279 mg
Total Fiber	1 g
Protein	17 g
Carbohydrates	7 g
Potassium	302 mg

Poached Salmon

The tomato relish adds just the right amount of flavor.

Spicy Tomato Relish
- 2 medium tomatoes, chopped
- 2 tablespoons yellow onion, finely chopped
- 2 tablespoons fresh parsley, finely chopped
- 1 teaspoon red pepper flakes, or to taste
- ¼ cup red wine vinegar
- 2 tablespoons olive oil
- black pepper, to taste

Salmon
- 4 5-ounce salmon steaks
- 3 cups water
- 4 black peppercorns
- 1 lemon, thickly sliced
- 3 parsley sprigs
- 1 small onion, thickly sliced
- 2 bay leaves

1. For relish, combine all the ingredients in a bowl and set aside.

2. Using a pan large enough to hold salmon steaks, bring water to a boil and add peppercorns, lemon slices, parsley, onion, and bay leaf.

3. Lower heat to a gentle simmer, cover, and let flavors infuse for 5 minutes. Add salmon steaks and make sure they are covered with water. Add additional water if needed.

4. Cook, uncovered, for 10 to 12 minutes or until fish is just tender. It will flake easily when tested with a fork. Never let water boil or fish will toughen.

5. Divide the relish on four plates.

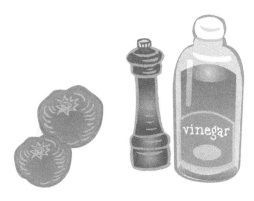

Yield:	4 servings
Serving size:	1 salmon steak and ¼ cup relish
Calories	246
Total Fat	10 g
Saturated Fat	3 g
Cholesterol	93 mg
Sodium	94 mg
Total Fiber	2 g
Protein	31 g
Carbohydrates	7 g
Potassium	945 mg

Jamaican Jerk Chicken

The spices and peppers in this dish will transport you to a whole new taste.

- ½ teaspoon cinnamon, ground
- 1½ teaspoons allspice, ground
- 1½ teaspoons black pepper, ground
- 1 tablespoon hot pepper, chopped
- 1 teaspoon hot pepper, crushed, dried
- 2 teaspoons oregano, crushed
- 2 teaspoons thyme, crushed
- ½ teaspoon salt
- 6 cloves garlic, finely chopped
- 1 cup onion, pureed or finely chopped
- ¼ cup vinegar
- 3 tablespoons brown sugar
- 8 pieces chicken, skinless (4 breasts, 4 drumsticks)

1. Preheat oven to 350 °F. Wash chicken and pat dry.

2. Combine all ingredients except chicken in large bowl. Rub seasonings over chicken and marinate in refrigerator for 6 hours or longer.

3. Space chicken evenly on nonstick or lightly greased baking pan.

4. Cover with aluminum foil and bake for 40 minutes. Remove foil and continue baking for an additional 30–40 minutes or until the meat can easily be pulled away from the bone with a fork.

Yield:	**10 servings**
Serving size:	**½ breast or 2 small drumsticks**
Calories	113
Total Fat	3 g
Saturated Fat	1 g
Cholesterol	49 mg
Sodium	161 mg
Total Fiber	1 g
Protein	16 g
Carbohydrates	6 g
Potassium	192 mg

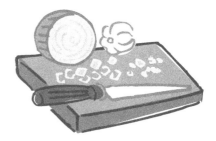

Baked Pork Chops

You can really sink your chops into these—they're made moist and spicy with egg whites, evaporated milk, and a lively blend of herbs.

- 6 lean center-cut pork chops, ½-inch thick
- 1 egg white
- 1 cup fat-free evaporated milk
- ¾ cup cornflake crumbs
- ¼ cup fine, dry bread crumbs
- 4 teaspoons paprika
- 2 teaspoons oregano
- ¾ teaspoon chili powder
- 2 teaspoons garlic powder
- 2 teaspoons black pepper
- ⅛ teaspoon cayenne pepper
- ⅛ teaspoon dry mustard
- 2 teaspoons salt
- nonstick cooking spray, as needed

1. Preheat oven to 375 °F.

2. Trim fat from pork chops.

3. Beat egg white with fat-free evaporated milk. Place pork chops in milk mixture and let stand for 5 minutes, turning once.

4. Meanwhile, mix cornflake crumbs, bread crumbs, spices, and salt in small bowl.

5. Use nonstick cooking spray on 13 x 9-inch baking pan.

6. Remove pork chops from milk mixture and coat thoroughly with crumb mixture.

7. Place pork chops in pan and bake for 20 minutes. Turn pork chops and bake for an additional 15 minutes or until no pink remains.

   Note: Try the recipe with skinless, boneless chicken or turkey parts or fish—bake for just 20 minutes.

Yield:	6 servings
Serving size:	1 pork chop
Calories	216
Total Fat	10 g
Saturated Fat	8 g
Cholesterol	62 mg
Sodium	346 mg
Total Fiber	1 g
Protein	25 g
Carbohydrates	10 g
Potassium	414 mg

Jumpin' Jambalaya

Here is a jambalaya that your family can enjoy. It has lots of flavor, veggies, and tasty low-fat meats! Green salad is a nice side dish.

- 14 ounces low-fat turkey kielbasa
- 1 pound boneless, skinless chicken breast
- nonstick cooking spray
- 1 medium celery stalk, chopped
- 2 small onions, chopped
- 4 cloves garlic, chopped
- 1 small bunch green onions, chopped
- 1 medium green bell pepper, chopped
- 1 14½-ounce can of diced tomatoes, no salt added
- 1½ cups uncooked brown rice
- 4 cups water
- 2 cubes, low-sodium chicken bouillon
- 1 bay leaf
- 1½ teaspoons cayenne pepper
- 3 tablespoons parsley, finely chopped

1. Wash chicken and pat dry. Cut the chicken breast and kielbasa into 1-inch chunks.

2. Spray a medium-sized pan with nonstick cooking spray. Brown the sausage and chicken over medium heat and remove from the pan.

3. Add next 6 ingredients to the same pot and cook over medium heat for 10 minutes.

Yield:	9 servings
Serving size:	**1 cup**
Calories	250
Total Fat	4 g
Saturated Fat	1 g
Cholesterol	53 mg
Sodium	531 mg
Total Fiber	5 g
Protein	22 g
Carbohydrates	31 g
Potassium	427 mg

4. Put the cooked meat back in the pot; add the rice, water, chicken bouillon cubes, bay leaf, and cayenne pepper. Bring to a boil. Cover, reduce heat, and let simmer for about 50 minutes* or until the water is evaporated.

5. Stir in parsley and serve warm.

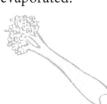

Instant brown rice will take less time.

Scrumptious Meat Loaf

Got the meat loaf blahs? This recipe transforms the ordinary into the extraordinary.

- 1 pound extra lean ground beef
- ½ cup tomato paste
- 4 cups onion, chopped
- 4 cups green pepper
- 4 cups red pepper
- 1 cup fresh tomatoes, blanched, chopped
- 2 teaspoons mustard, low sodium
- 4 teaspoons ground black pepper
- 2 teaspoons hot pepper, chopped
- 2 cloves garlic, chopped
- 2 scallions, chopped
- 2 teaspoons ground ginger
- 8 teaspoons ground nutmeg
- 1 teaspoon orange rind, grated
- 2 teaspoons thyme, crushed
- 4 cups bread crumbs, finely grated

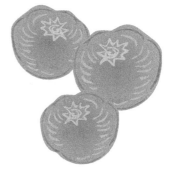

1. Preheat oven to 350 °F.

2. Mix all ingredients together.

3. Place in 1-pound loaf pan (preferably with drip rack) and bake, covered, for 50 minutes.

4. Uncover pan and continue baking for 12 minutes.

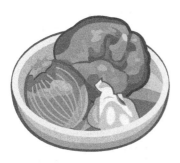

Yield:	6 servings
Serving size:	1¼-inch-thick slice
Calories	193
Total Fat	9 g
Saturated Fat	3 g
Cholesterol	45 mg
Sodium	91 mg
Total Fiber	2 g
Protein	17 g
Carbohydrates	11 g
Potassium	513 mg

Spicy Southern Barbecued Chicken

Let yourself fall under the spell of this Southern-style, sweet barbecue sauce.

- 5 tablespoons tomato paste
- 1 teaspoon ketchup
- 2 teaspoons honey
- 1 teaspoon molasses
- 1 teaspoon Worcestershire sauce
- 4 teaspoons white vinegar
- ¾ teaspoon cayenne pepper
- ⅛ teaspoon black pepper
- ¼ teaspoon onion powder
- 2 cloves garlic, minced
- ⅛ teaspoon ginger, grated
- 1½ pounds chicken (breasts, drumsticks), skinless

1. Combine all ingredients except chicken in saucepan.

2. Simmer for 15 minutes.

3. Wash chicken and pat dry. Place it on large platter and brush with half the sauce mixture.

4. Cover with plastic wrap and marinate in refrigerator for 1 hour.

5. Place chicken on baking sheet lined with aluminum foil and broil for 10 minutes on each side to seal in juices.

6. Remove from broiler and add remaining sauce to chicken. Cover with aluminum foil and bake at 350 °F for 30 minutes.

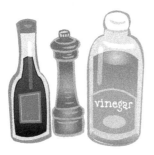

Yield:	6 servings
Serving size:	½ breast or 2 small drumsticks
Calories	176
Total Fat	4 g
Saturated Fat	0 g
Cholesterol	81 mg
Sodium	199 mg
Total Fiber	1 g
Protein	27 g
Carbohydrates	7 g
Potassium	392 mg

Desserts

1-2-3 Peach Cobbler

Mock-Southern Sweet Potato Pie

Southern Banana Pudding

Summer Breeze Smoothie

Tangy Fruit Salad

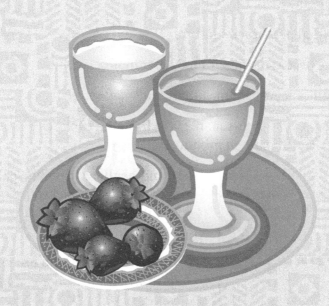

1-2-3 Peach Cobbler

What could be better than peach cobbler straight from the oven?
Try this healthier version of the classic favorite.

- ½ teaspoon ground cinnamon
- 1 tablespoon vanilla extract
- 2 tablespoons cornstarch
- 1 cup peach nectar
- ¼ cup pineapple juice or peach juice (if desired, use juice reserved from canned peaches)
- 2 16-ounce cans of peaches, packed in juice, drained, (or 1¾ pounds, fresh, sliced)

- 1 tablespoon tub margarine
- 1 cup dry pancake mix
- ⅔ cup all-purpose flour
- ½ cup sugar
- ⅔ cup fat-free evaporated milk
- ½ teaspoon nutmeg
- 1 tablespoon brown sugar
- nonstick cooking spray, as needed

1. Preheat oven to 400 °F.

2. Combine cinnamon, vanilla, cornstarch, peach nectar, and juice in saucepan over medium heat. Stir constantly until mixture thickens and bubbles.

3. Add sliced peaches to mixture.

4. Reduce heat and simmer for 5–10 minutes.

5. In another saucepan, melt margarine and set aside.

6. Lightly spray 8-inch-square glass dish with cooking spray. Pour hot peach mixture into dish.

Yield:	8 servings
Serving size:	1 square
Calories	271
Total Fat	4 g
Saturated Fat	0 g
Cholesterol	0 mg
Sodium	263 mg
Total Fiber	2 g
Protein	4 g
Carbohydrates	54 g
Potassium	284 mg

7. In another bowl, combine pancake mix, flour, sugar, and melted margarine. Stir in milk. Quickly spoon this mixture over peach mixture.

8. Combine nutmeg and brown sugar. Sprinkle mixture on top of batter.

9. Bake for 15–20 minutes or until golden brown.

10. Cool and cut into eight squares.

Mock-Southern Sweet Potato Pie

There's nothing fake about the flavor in this heart healthy treat.

Crust

- 1¼ cups flour
- ¼ teaspoon sugar
- ⅓ cup fat-free milk
- 2 tablespoons vegetable oil

Filling

- ¼ cup white sugar
- ¼ cup brown sugar
- ½ teaspoon salt
- ¼ teaspoon nutmeg
- 3 large eggs, beaten
- ¼ cup fat-free evaporated milk
- 1 teaspoon vanilla extract
- 3 cups sweet potatoes (cooked and mashed)

1. Preheat oven to 350 °F.

To prepare crust:

2. Combine flour and sugar in bowl.

3. Add milk and oil to flour mixture.

4. Stir with fork until well mixed. Form pastry into smooth ball with your hands.

5. Roll ball between two 12-inch squares of wax paper, using short, brisk strokes, until pastry reaches edges of paper.

6. Peel off top paper and invert crust into pie plate.

To prepare filling:

7. Combine sugars, salt, nutmeg, and eggs.

8. Add milk and vanilla. Stir.

9. Add sweet potatoes and mix well.

Putting it together:

10. Pour mixture into pie shell.

11. Bake for 60 minutes or until crust is golden brown. Cool and cut into 16 slices.

Yield:	16 servings
Serving size:	1 slice
Calories	147
Total Fat	3 g
Saturated Fat	1 g
Cholesterol	40 mg
Sodium	98 mg
Total Fiber	2 g
Protein	4 g
Carbohydrates	27 g
Potassium	293 mg

Southern Banana Pudding

This traditional dessert with a healthy twist will please your entire family.

- 3¾ cups cold, fat-free milk
- 2 small packages (4 serving size) of fat-free, sugar-free instant vanilla pudding and pie-filling mix
- 32 reduced-fat vanilla wafers
- 2 medium bananas, sliced
- 2 cups fat-free, frozen whipped topping, thawed

1. Mix 3½ cups of the milk with the pudding mixes. Beat the pudding mixture with a wire whisk for 2 minutes until it is well blended. Let stand for 5 minutes.

2. Fold 1 cup of the whipped topping into the pudding mix.

3. Arrange a layer of wafers on the bottom and sides of a 2-quart serving bowl. Drizzle 2 tablespoons of the remaining milk over the wafers. Add a layer of banana slices and top with one-third of the pudding.

4. Repeat layers, drizzling wafer layer with remaining milk and ending with pudding. Spread the remaining whipped topping over the pudding.

5. Refrigerate for at least 3 hours before serving.

Yield:	10 servings
Serving size:	¾ cup
Calories	143
Total Fat	2 g
Saturated Fat	1 g
Cholesterol	2 mg
Sodium	329 mg
Total Fiber	1 g
Protein	4 g
Carbohydrates	29 g
Potassium	237 mg

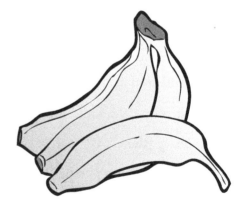

Summer Breeze Smoothie

Here's a perfect low-fat thirst quencher.

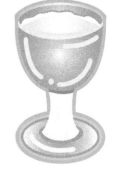

- 1 cup yogurt, plain, nonfat
- 6 medium strawberries
- 1 cup pineapple, crushed, canned in juice
- 1 medium banana
- 1 teaspoon vanilla extract
- 4 ice cubes

1. Place all ingredients in blender and puree until smooth.

2. Serve in frosted glass.

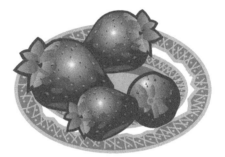

Yield:	3 servings
Serving size:	**1 cup**
Calories	121
Total Fat	0 g
Saturated Fat	0 g
Cholesterol	1 mg
Sodium	64 mg
Total Fiber	2 g
Protein	6 g
Carbohydrates	24 g
Potassium	483 mg

Tangy Fruit Salad

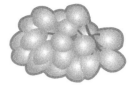

What a great way to enjoy fruit!

- 2 tablespoons instant sugar-free vanilla pudding mix*
- 1 cup light vanilla yogurt
- 1 15-ounce can pineapple chunks, in juice, drained
- 1 11-ounce can mandarin oranges, in juice, drained
- 1 cup grapes
- 2 medium bananas, sliced

1. Combine pudding mix and yogurt. Mix fruit in medium bowl.

2. Stir fruit into yogurt mixture.

3. Refrigerate. Serve when chilled.

* **The leftover pudding mix can be blended with milk (according to the box instructions) and used as a topping for berries.**

Yield:	6 servings
Serving size:	½ cup
Calories	134
Total Fat	0 g
Saturated Fat	0 g
Cholesterol	1 mg
Sodium	38 mg
Total Fiber	3 g
Protein	3 g
Carbohydrates	33 g
Potassium	417 mg

Recipe Substitutions for Heart Healthy Cooking

Is It Done Yet? Temperature Rules for Safe Cooking

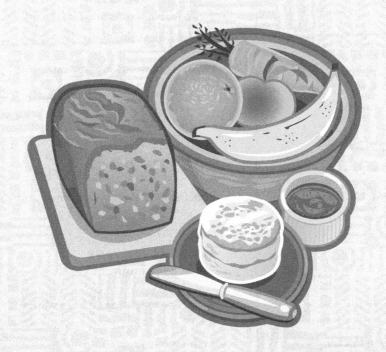

Recipe Substitutions for Heart Healthy Cooking

Use the suggestions below to lower saturated fat and calories in your favorite recipes. Add herbs and spices instead of salt to enhance flavor.

Recipe calls for:	Substitute:
Whole milk	• Fat-free or low-fat (1%) milk
Cream	• Evaporated fat-free milk • Mix equal amounts low-fat (1%) milk and fat-free evaporated milk
Sour cream	• Fat-free or low-fat sour cream
Mayonnaise	• Fat-free or low-fat mayonnaise
1 cup of butter	• 1 cup tub margarine • ⅔ cup vegetable oil
Oil (for baking)	• Equal amounts of applesauce or prune puree
Oil (for sauteing)	• Water • Nonstick cooking spray • Low-sodium broth
1 whole egg	• ¼ cup egg substitute or 2 egg whites
1 egg to thicken	• 1 tablespoon flour
Ground beef (all types)	• Extra lean ground beef or turkey (10% or less fat) • Turkey (10% or less fat)

Recipe calls for:	Substitute:
Sausage	• Turkey sausage (10% or less fat) • Vegetarian sausage
Salad dressing	• Fat-free or low-fat dressing • Flavored vinaigrette • Flavored vinaigrette (made with olive oil, water and vinegar, or lemon juice)
Cream soup	• Fat-free or low-fat canned cream soup • Homemade broth after removing the fat • Fat-free broth mixed with fat-free milk or fat-free evaporated milk

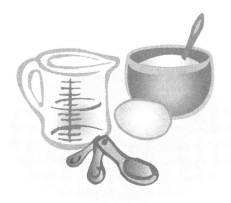

Is It Done Yet?
Temperature Rules for Safe Cooking

Make sure you cook and keep foods at the correct temperature to ensure food safety. Bacteria can grow in foods between 40 °F and 140 °F. To keep foods out of this danger zone, keep cold foods cold and hot foods hot. Use a clean thermometer and measure the internal temperature of cooked food to make sure meat, poultry, and egg dishes are cooked to the temperatures listed below.

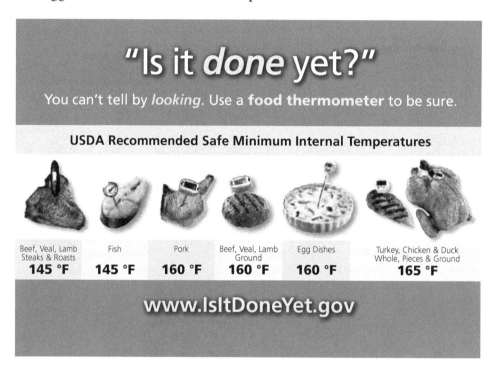

"Is it *done* yet?"

You can't tell by *looking*. Use a **food thermometer** to be sure.

USDA Recommended Safe Minimum Internal Temperatures

Beef, Veal, Lamb Steaks & Roasts	Fish	Pork	Beef, Veal, Lamb Ground	Egg Dishes	Turkey, Chicken & Duck Whole, Pieces & Ground
145 °F	**145 °F**	**160 °F**	**160 °F**	**160 °F**	**165 °F**

www.IsItDoneYet.gov

DISCRIMINATION PROHIBITED: Under provisions of applicable public laws enacted by Congress since 1964, no person in the United States shall, on the grounds of race, color, national origin, handicap, or age, be excluded from participation in, be denied the benefits of, or be subjected to discrimination under any program or activity (or, on the basis of sex, with respect to any education program or activity) receiving Federal financial assistance. In addition, Executive Order 11141 prohibits discrimination on the basis of age by contractors and subcontractors in the performance of Federal contracts, and Executive Order 11246 states that no federally funded contractor may discriminate against any employee or applicant for employment because of race, color, religion, sex, or national origin. Therefore, the National Heart, Lung, and Blood Institute must be operated in compliance with these laws and Executive Orders.

CPSIA information can be obtained
at www.ICGtesting.com
Printed in the USA
BVHW010559120320
574765BV00001B/21

9 781782 660736